ABOUT FASTING

by

OTTO H. F. BUCHINGER, M.D.

Translated from the German by
GEOFFREY A. DUDLEY, B.A.

THORSONS PUBLISHERS LIMITED
Wellingborough, Northamptonshire

First published 1961
Ninth Impression 1977
Tenth Impression 1980

PUBLISHER'S NOTE

It is pointed out that the procedures outlined in the second section of this book (page 35) are those applying on the Continent in connection with the fasting sanatoria operating there.

These procedures need not necessarily apply in relation to fasting therapy as prescribed by practitioners in this country.

ISBN 0 7225 0075 0

Printed and bound in Great Britain by
Hunt Barnard Printing Ltd., Aylesbury, Bucks

CONTENTS

FOREWORD

THIS little book[1] is addressed to the intelligent layman, to the sick and the healthy—or to those who are still healthy. It seeks in a simple way to spread the profound truth of the healing fast even where a knowledge of technical terms cannot be taken for granted. On the other hand it is impossible here to give individual questions specialised treatment. For this purpose it would be necessary to consult the literature of fasting.

The question of the "how" of healing by fasting is basically difficult to answer. Every era—according to the state of its knowledge—sets up different explanations and theories. However, having convinced oneself that fasting sets free, mobilises and brings to bear the body's self-healing powers (the "physician within," the "Archaeus" of Paracelsus), one can certainly have confidence in this method of treatment.

Fasting is, in fact, an ideal method of treatment for the whole being. In this book there rings out a new small voice in the great chorus of those who in an outspokenly scientific way recommend fasting for what it really is—*a royal road to healing* for anyone who agrees to take it for the recovery and regeneration of body, mind and spirit.

Bad Pyrmont.   OTTO H. F. BUCHINGER.

---

[1] Dr. med. Otto H. F. Buchinger: *Gesund werden—gesund bleiben durch die Heilfastenkur* (Bruno Wilkens Verlag, Hanover), of which the present translation is an abridged version.

PART ONE

FASTING AND DISEASE

CHAPTER ONE

HOW DID I FALL ILL?

AFTER times of privation and catastrophe such as the war and postwar years little sympathy will be found for fasting—especially if fasting is inappropriately equated with hunger. People think with alarm of the results of lack of nourishment and undernourishment. But we can easily show that many more people become ill at full tables (even suffering, indeed, from lack of nourishment and undernourishment) than in times of food shortage. Scarce and restricted food with darker (wholemeal) bread reduces the frequency of chronic constipation, which is so widespread. Appendicitis, diabetes and other diseases fall off in number, and heart, circulatory, rheumatic as well as many stomach, intestinal, kidney and nerve complaints lessen as a person's weight comes down. A fattening diet wrong in quality and quantity and wrongly prepared turns a blessing into a curse and an affliction. A surprisingly high percentage of all diseases originates from that kind of wrong nourishment. Practically every doctor knows from experience that a substantial part of his patients is recruited from the victims of improper diet, overnourishment, tobacco and alcohol !

From ordinary plain cooking we can get much pleasure and enjoyment—but also much distress, if we continue to make certain mistakes. The Swiss physician Bircher-Benner has explained and demonstrated to us that "Eating and drinking keep body and soul together" must read "Moderate and healthy eating and drinking can keep body and soul together." We add : especially if—following the rhythm of nature—we purify ourselves by fasting once a year for the prevention of illness. How wrong is the view, which is met both in home

and hospital catering, that the body must have a fattening
over-supply of nourishment to strengthen its defences and
build up its powers of resistance. This elementary error
evidently springs from the economic way of thinking ("Save
for a rainy day"); it treats people like the pig, the "farmer's
money-box," and this wrong attitude takes its revenge in a
tragic manner. Not only a whole host of diseases like rheumatism, gout, eczema, etc., but even cancer can then visit us like
a bolt from the blue. We know that—in the long run—fat,
stout, overfed people are much more susceptible to illness,
have less stamina and more often become casualties than slim,
tough and resistant people who know the secret of a plain,
wholesome and sparing vegetarian diet, the full value of which
is obtained by chewing it well.

The devil (in whom the educated do not believe) has perverted the blessings of civilisation into their opposite. Pro-
fessional practice, time and technology have us in their grasp,
ruling and driving us. We are past masters of artificial activi-
ties, but the natural functions of our body lie deeper. The
processes of metabolism have been slowed down or entirely
checked. Next to the influences of living in a nervous, anxious,
cramped or anger-ridden atmosphere, overfeeding and wrong
feeding, too little exercise as well as tobacco and alcohol contribute decisively to all kinds of diseases and sufferings. The
organism's many possibilities of helping itself without an illness
becoming manifest and of putting itself in order again are
sooner or later exhausted. The body's processes of combustion and energy-transformation degenerate. Changes occur
in the fine blood vessels (capillaries) and there are general or
local disturbances of circulation. The harmonious working
together of all organs, parts, tissues and glands is upset. We
are taken unawares by suddenly receiving a surprise packet of
ills. Toxic substances have found their way into the body.
Fatigue, headaches, excess of uric acid and rheumatic poisons,
abdominal distention, feelings of anxiety and oppression of the
heart and lungs announce themselves. The poisons of metabolism are deposited in numerous tissues, organs and joints,
spreading infections. A human wreck, pain-ridden, suffering,

tired of life, often with fatty degeneration as well, is the result.

How many of us know the beginnings and all the causal connections? In explaining his "eightfold path," Buddha says : "The sufferings which overtake man are the fruit of his desires." We add : the fruit of his mistakes, of his omissions! Frequently we hear that knowledge is power. No doubt there is something in that. We must once again learn to have the courage to protest against food which is wrong in quality and quantity, against the pernicious habits of smoking and drinking, against the spoiling of food by industrial processes. We have, of course, seen that it is a many-sided problem. We started off by considering the beneficial` effect of a sparing diet. The restricted consumption of· tobacco and alcohol in times of privation also contributes to the reduction of diseases of the heart, circulation, stomach, intestine and nerves. We must clearly impress it upon ourselves that man with his body is subject to the laws of nature. The sum total of the mistakes we make with nutrition, tobacco, alcohol, spoilt and impoverished food containing artificial colouring matter, etc., goes on our bill of health. Often out of a clear blue sky we suddenly experience the ruin of our health and working efficiency in the form of serious, acute, or chronic disease. In this state the time has come for fasting.

In acute cases of illness, however, we receive a warning sign from nature : one of the first symptoms of the onset of an acute disease is loss of appetite.

Therefore, here again, too, fasting is characterised as a healing measure of nature. Today it has again become clear to medical science that in falling ill the organism with its complaints and symptoms (loss of appetite, sweating, diarrhoea, vomiting, etc.) makes explicit as a rule its own healing measures. I call to mind at this point the special assessment of fever as a healing fever, the remedial suppression of which by tablets and ice-bags is very often a technical mistake. As Nietzsche put it : "There is more sense in your body than in your will." The mistake of feeding a patient on a fattening diet, like immoderate eating and drinking in general, encases the heart, intestines, liver (the most important organ of metabolism) and in the end the whole body in an armour of fat which banishes joy of life, capacity for work and health. The "physician within," as the famous, gallant and much-travelled physician Paracelsus von Hohenheim nearly five hundred years ago called the wise self-healing power, has command of abilities without which even the most practised doctor could not perform any healing art. Today, of course, in acute diseases, like scarlet fever, tonsillitis, diphtheria, pneumonia, influenza, etc., the patient is allowed to fast with a good evacuation of the bowels and a drink of fruit juice or tea. How much more, however, does this understanding need to be extended to the harder task of shifting chronic diseases? We shall speak in detail about that later.

But we have forgotten what is quite essential: does man consist only of the body? According to the many newspaper articles and reports of conferences, it is almost to be regarded as an old, newly-discovered truth that the spiritual person-ality of man which dwells in our bodily frame is of immortal origin and controls the delicate mechanism of our manifold physical, nervous, metabolic and hormonal functions. All modern and well-founded results of investigation (Carl du Prel, Coué, Ricker, Speransky, also the American parapsy-chologist Rhine) see the origin of disease in a disharmony of mind and spirit. The faulty tension in this creative central layer of existence makes itself felt like an interruption in the telephone service. Now some or at least several of the sub-scribers are disturbed or even at times disconnected. Even infections do not get a hold unless susceptibility to disease meets them half way on a nutritional basis. What is the only thing left for man to do in this situation? Bircher-Benner speaks of the laws of life, for violation of which nature con-sistently punishes us with disease. And the biologist Dr. Her-bert Fritsche says : "The advice which medical science can give to a patient is always : Do all you can to fulfil the laws which you have infringed. To make that possible, undergo for once a thorough cleansing. . . ."

Thus we now see ourselves facing a challenge : to purify the body by fasting, to build it up again—but at the same time also to tighten and restore the power lines of the spirit. This active striving for reunion and the reconciliation of the spiritual personality of man with the material body in which it dwells and with the God of revelation is called in Latin "religio." It is no wonder, then, that during the five thousand odd years of mankind's history which today we can survey, fasting represented in all ages and climes a way of healing and sanctification of far-reaching importance. The religious fast which we find in all the higher religions of mankind served at the same time to preserve the health of the body, the temple of the immortal soul. Greatly to the loss of sick humanity, the healing fast was overlooked by medicine during the many decades of scientific-materialistic thought. Newly discovered at the turn of the century, it has today regained a worthy position as a royal road of healing.

CHAPTER TWO

WHEN IS FASTING NECESSARY?

No doubt many of my readers know the anecdote of the surgeon who divided all people into two groups, those who allow themselves to be operated on and those who don't. The fasting specialist, too, could be similarly disposed to assess people. He has lived to see growing numbers of successes from the healing fast under experienced medical direction. Humbly and fully convinced, he bows to the wisdom and power of the "physician within" and of our body's natural self-healing effort which has been liberated in the fast. He bows to these healing powers, whose action he may set in motion and pilot for the benefit of sick people.

If we now ask the doctor about the indications for applying his treatment, he will say that for him there are basically two main groups of diseases: those in which one must fast and those in which one may fast. How are we to understand

that? It is not at all hard to imagine diseases for the successful treatment of which we must fast. But there are also conditions of susceptibility to disease which are smouldering in
readiness to break out but still not always recognisable. Those
are the diseases in which one *may* fast and often *should*!

The preventive fast! Following the rhythm of nature, this
takes place every year in the spring, as a spring-clean, so to
speak, to remove accumulated impurities.

A general view of the diagnostic pictures in which one can
or—better still—should fast is to be gained as follows :

1. The sphere of disorders of *metabolism* like obesity and
chronic underweight, rheumatism in the joints and muscles,
sciatica, diabetes in the initial stages before it is too far
advanced.

2. The sphere of *diseases of the heart, circulation and blood
vessels*, such as angina pectoris, coronary thrombosis, high or
low blood pressure, congestions in the blood stream and lymphatic system, hot flushes, plethora, after-effects of phlebitis
and thrombosis, disturbances of circulation, early cases of
arteriosclerosis, many symptoms of ageing, vascular constrictions with gangrene of the toes, etc.

3. The so-called *"executive's disease."* (Note the detailed
review in Chapter Five.)

4. *Blood changes* which have arisen from all sorts of
disease influences, as, for example, from chronic inflammation or suppuration of the tonsils or the roots of the teeth,
from chronic suppuration of the middle ear, plethora and tendency to bleed in consequence of poisoning; results of abuse of
nicotine, alcohol, arsenic, bismuth, mercury, morphia, sleep-
ing pills and remedies generally, as far as these effects are not
yet too advanced.

5. *Skin diseases* like psoriasis, eczema, nettlerash, oversensi-
tive skins, and a tendency to ulcers, acne, boils and erysipelas.

6. *Diseases of the digestive organs,* catarrh of the stomach
and bowels, loss of appetite, liver and gall-bladder diseases,
stubborn constipation, a tendency to diarrhoea, relaxed
bowels and—but only seldom—formation of ulcers in the
stomach and bowels.

7. *Diseases of the respiratory organs,* chronic catarrh of throat, chest and nose, slight chills, bronchial asthma, and after-effects of attacks of pneumonia and non-tuberculosis pleurisy.

8. *Kidney and bladder diseases,* such as nephritis and pyelitis, vesical and renal calculus and haemorrhage, and renal atrophy if not too far advanced.

9. *Female complaints,* like menopausal symptoms, chronic inflammations of the womb, Fallopian tube and ovary, benign tumours of the female sex organs, disturbances of the menstrual flow (in regularity, strength, duration, painfulness), vomiting in pregnancy and tendency to miscarriage.

10. *Allergies,* as, for example, hay fever, idiosyncrasies, which can show themselves in many kinds of reactions in very many parts and organs of the body. Only the site of the allergic reaction, however, is improved.

11. *Conditions following venereal diseases* or their intensive treatment.

12. *Nervous complaints* (but no insane or psychopaths!), such as nervous exhaustion, weakness of convalescence, migraine, recurring headache, neuralgia, neuritis, insomnia, nervous disturbances of various kinds, occupational and emotional inhibitions, depression, sexual weakness or over-stimulation.

13. The many forms of *glandular disturbances* (ovaries, etc.) we can also mention here, likewise, too, the many pictures of thyroid-gland deficiency, because both these groups frequently derive from a disturbance of the vegetative nervous system, which is quite commonly an indication for curative fasting.

14. *Latent susceptibility to cancer,* in which the question is one of prevention.

15. *Eye diseases* like chronic iritis, retinitis, and many in-flammatory processes of the eyes generally—also in sporadic cases of glaucoma—respond favourably to fasting. During the treatment, however, they need a specialist's supervision.

16. *Parodontal diseases.*

17. Fasting in readiness for operations and for better and easier recovery afterwards.

18. Diseased conditions which have had their origin in under-nutrition and malnutrition.

19. Spring fevers and fatigue.

After this summary it seems desirable to discuss one or two groups of diseases. Let us begin with the various aspects of the *obesity* group.

CHAPTER THREE

OVERWEIGHT AND RHEUMATISM

WHAT are the causes of *overweight*? Essentially we can distinguish three groups of causes :

A. Lazy elimination by the bowels, kidneys and skin. At the root of it there probably lie reduced combustion processes in metabolism.

B. Particular glands, groups of glands or the whole *hormonal action collectively run off the rails* (pituitary gland, thyroid gland, adrenal gland, ovaries, testes, vegetative midbrain centre and others). Hormonally-conditioned obesity following pregnancy is much rarer than we are generally inclined to suppose. This form of obesity often arises from a mode of living and eating which in quality and quantity is unsuitable for pregnant women and nursing mothers. How many become ill and fat less through the meals themselves than through the "in-between" snacks of cakes, drinking chocolate and chocolates, and the extra physical inertia !

More than half of all cases of heart disease (especially among older people) are the result of overweight. According to life insurance statistics, overweight increases the mortality rate. A person who weighs 10 per cent more than he should, has, according to probability calculations, about a 20 per cent shorter life-expectation than the person of normal weight, given the same standard of health. Even if he weighs only 20 per cent more, he has a life-expectation shortened by about 40 per cent, and so on.[1]

C. *Mixed causes of obesity.* Disturbances of the body's economy resulting from faulty metabolism of fat in young girls, in women during the climacteric, in men and women in prison (lipodystrophy), from food too rich in water and carbohydrate content and long-standingly too poor in protein. Disturbances of the water economy, and the like.

As we see, these are disease conditions which require prompt correction—but I am now asked: how can overweight endanger the heart and circulation, which would adjust themselves to meet the increased demand? The answer can only be that the heart and circulation of an overweight person become disordered *because* they try to adapt themselves to the increased demand. Let them fail to do this and the chapter is closed with an early breakdown. It is typical of our time that we can get a better understanding if we take an example from the mechanical field. I can "tune up" the engine of a private car until it is like the engine of a motor lorry. I bring the machine to a higher performance when I raise its number of revolutions. The heart reacts in exactly the same way: if it has more weight to carry it increases the pulse rate and blood pressure.

Now we understand just how the lives of those who are overweight—even the non-smokers among them—are in danger and hang on a heartbeat. But we also understand just why overweight people must undergo regularly repeated fasts and make up their minds to avoid in their food and way of life (e.g. lack of exercise, shallow breathing) everything that could contribute to the continuation of the trouble.

But *much* more frequently we doctors diagnose high blood pressure *and* overweight, angina pectoris *and* overweight, severe rheumatism *and* overweight, skin and other diseases

[1] The "correct" body weight for the individual is, according to Dr. Träbert, most conveniently reckoned with the "Individual Weight Correlator" from the height, chest measurement and age. If—as was once the practice—the weight is worked out by rule of thumb, it gives false results.

and overweight, and so on. In short, disease *plus* overweight is incidental to repeated treatments especially where the specialist in fasting is concerned. The customary use of purgatives is not suitable for losing weight, but only for causing injury to the intestinal area, and the peristaltic movement, and for disturbing the calcium content of the blood.

In the body showing fatty degeneration the tissues contain less water than do those of a patient whose water economy is disturbed. So the unhealthily fat must fast longer than those who have merely put on weight, for large deposits of fat give way only to the assault of long and consistent fasting. In these cases, too, the training for a rational manner of living and eating after the fast is particularly important. Annual repetitions of the fast are not to be avoided.

It is only too easy to see that *health fasting* as a—let us say —heroic method of treatment *makes considerable demands on the intelligence, will and character of the fasting person.* "Wash me but don't make my skin wet!" is a dangerous maxim. Only exact observance of the inner and outer discipline of fasting can bring the desired help. Even if we bear in mind that the healing fast alone can help towards *getting* well, it later rests on what the patient himself does and allows whether he *remains* well. We then acknowledge the uninterrupted sacrifices of the pleasures of the table which we have to make in quantity and quality—if we are serious about good health. One or other of us is already giving up at that point and thinking that he can go an easier, much publicised and up-to-date way which comes from the U.S.A. and has to do with calculations and juggling with calories. Less carbohydrates and more protein are recommended (plenty of eggs, meat and coffee each day). The outcome is held to be a reduction of weight by limiting the useful calories. This does not let a person feel hungry and so enables him to slim effortlessly—but at the same time it makes him ill or lays the foundation for his becoming ill. For the tremendous overfeeding with meat, eggs, coffee and other uric acid-forming agents brings with it in this apparently more comfortable way an excess of uric acid and an early harvest of those who are ripe for doctors, sanatoria or hospitals for slimming fanatics! This general state of impurity must in the end bring with it rheumatism, gout and other afflictions.

The final result is that the wiser among these deceived and self-deceiving persons will after that still decide for himself in favour of fasting as a convert!

The most surprising of the many fashionable books on slimming and rejuvenation is that of Cooley, who maintains that the reason why slimness cannot be satisfactorily attained by fasting methods is that the fasting organism jealously holds on to its stores of fat right to the bitter end. Exactly the opposite, however, proves to be the case!

The same can be said about the many kinds of *slimming pills*. Beware of a disturbance of the finely-balanced hormone economy by slimming hormones and thyroid extracts. Hormonal chaos is very easily brought on. Nor does the organism let itself be outwitted by this or that slimming sugar or chemical remedy. Simple as it looks on paper ("Take it and there you are"), it isn't really. Our body is not a retort in which a convenient chemical slimming reaction can take place. Unpleasant after-effects and side-reactions are to be feared, e.g. in metabolism. The living structure of the mysterious play of energy and metabolism is not to be disturbed with dead but active chemical material, even if it is only a question of small quantities. It is only seldom that ways which fall in with our leaning to convenience are ways of health! Fasting is by no means a comfortable way, but it is certainly the most successful!

We have already touched upon the fact that we less often meet with fat people whose affliction may be said to be due to a *single* cause. Much more often we see *mixed forms of symptoms*. All types of obesity not only can but *should* fast! For the waste products and stores of fat are then broken down, burnt up and eliminated; and central disturbances (glands, water economy, etc.) are again regulated on normal healthy lines. In the true pituitary form we can occasionally bring about a healthy change with a hormone injection.

The person whose obesity is due to overeating, however, often finds it hard to fast—because in this case the fondness for food has usually gained the victory over the controlling, inhibiting instinct. If the taking of food which is wrong in quantity and quality has perverted not only the instinct but also the intelligence and will-power, then patient and doctor are going to take little pleasure in this treatment. Fasting calls for consistency and strength of will. Fat and bloated, lazy and averse to healthy physical exertion (for example, hiking, or at least walking!), disinclined, suspicious of all demands on character and personality—such patients want to be put through the treatment by the doctor, as it were, without having to take even the least active part mentally and physically. Although the doctor takes the greatest pains to guide them, they disclaim all effort of their own; yet as soon as any complaints break out, how they are wont to make themselves out to be healing and purifying crises! It is in line with their mental inertia that they prefer to go to the cinema than to their physician's evening health instruction. For of course the lectures too make demands!

The *habitual big eaters* also form the group of those who—mostly unknown to anyone—sabotage with sweets "under the counter" or normal taking of food in cafés the treatment which they have already successfully begun and so try to take in their doctor.

The doctor cannot *compel* his patient. But even in the most difficult cases a strong personality almost always succeeds in getting the sick person to carry out his treatment in a disciplined way and to complete it successfully. Indeed, patients who at first are unpromising often pull themselves together in the course of treatment, so that full of enthusiasm, they ask for the treatment to be extended. They even make up their minds to regulate their mode of living and eating at home—to the great joy of their doctor! The best of these patients come year after year.

After this discussion on the topic of "Fasting and fatness" the objection may be raised that *the effect of fasting on obesity can be understood, but not on thinness!* That, however, is only an apparent contradiction. The fasting treatment acts like a correct distribution of the load—the more a person has the more he can give away. Yet it is true that anyone who is underweight will lose a little more while fasting, but after a rationally controlled building-up diet he will end up heavier than he began.

That is confirmed by experiments with pigeons, cocks and newts (van Seeland, Morgulis). The increase in weight amounted on the average to 20 per cent of the original weight. The organism of thin, underweight people who are healthy is fundamentally cleared and regenerated in the fast. Naturally the applicant's suitability for treatment must be looked into beforehand in such cases. In the case of thinness several fasting efforts in succession are almost always preferable to one long fast.

Obesity is often linked with rheumatic complaints, which are of predominantly static origin and, as may be imagined, react well to the fasting treatment. *Rheumatic conditions* of the musculature and its surrounding sheaths and membranes respond best. I must here emphasise an important point : not only in heart and kidney diseases but in all forms of rheumatism the possibility of a stealthy, painless *slow poisoning by a focus of infection* must always be taken into account. This can come from the inflamed root of a dead tooth, or chronically inflamed tonsils, sinuses or gall-bladder. (If for no apparent reason the temperature goes up during the fast, the fasting director will think especially of such hidden foci of inflammation.)

Occasionally a chronically inflamed, smouldering appendix is shown to be the cause.

Unfortunately, if a rheumatic person's teeth, tonsils, appendix and perhaps his gall-bladder, too, are removed by operation, it turns out that the intestines with their flora of bacteria are to blame.

Basically a clearing-up of all foci of infection is desirable before treatment starts.

The weak musculature of the abdomen and intestinal wall must be strengthened by gymnastics and massage, and the rectum made firmer by purging. Diaphragms displaced by the blown-up stomach are lowered by intensive breathing exercises, and the heart relieved of its load. In suitable cases the success of the fast can be reinforced by Sauna baths, which secrete more moisture *via* the skin than *via* the kidneys.

We have already commented that muscular rheumatism reacts favourably to fasting. Not only it, but almost all *forms of chronic articular rheumatism and pains in the joints accompanying the menopause* respond with gratitude to the treatment, especially if the patient undergoes it year after year. For this annual repetition strengthens and deepens the good result. Of course, we must reserve judgment on those patients who are already confined to bed. Gout, too, gives both patient and doctor a hard nut to crack—especially in its severe form.

Where rheumatism is concerned, homoeopathy, hot mud and clay packs, massage and exercise often give excellent support to the main treatment, which is concluded with the prescription of a special diet of uncooked food and proper physical exercise.

In tuberculous arthritis one will, in most cases, advise against the fasting treatment. (A mountain climate, sunshine and a special diet are preferable to fasting in such a case.)

We gather from the Press that there are at least 95 million rheumatism sufferers in the world. Rheumatism research institutes, clinics, baths and specialists are continually at work. Victims of sciatica form a sizeable percentage of the pain-ridden army of the rheumatic. The fasting treatment can at last help many of them—often after fruitlessly trying other methods. We must draw the line, however, at the stubborn form of sciatica which comes from a slipped disc. Here fasting will afford only a brief improvement during the treatment. If special orthopaedic treatment cannot get rid of the trouble, then in the end surgery is all the more likely to succeed.

It is a source of surprise and delight to find how well *diabetics* generally succeed in standing a somewhat long fast. Of course, seriously ill patients accustomed to rather large quantities of insulin and greatly emaciated are no longer suitable for the treatment, but less seriously ill ones are. In fasting the excretion of sugar and acetone in the urine is reduced. Thirst and dryness of the mouth as well as restlessness, itching and physical weakness abate. In the course of fasting we hardly ever need to give insulin. After the treatment we almost always notice a reduced requirement of insulin and a better tolerance of carbohydrate.

CHAPTER FOUR

HEART AND CIRCULATORY DISORDERS

THE results of remedial fasting are really outstanding in most heart and circulatory disorders. This chapter is devoted to such disorders, arteriosclerosis and apoplectic seizure. Yet it would be incomplete if we did not also deal with *cardiac infarction*. We note with dismay the increasing number of tragic deaths caused by it. Talented (but overworked) executives, politicians, heads of industry and fashion kings, apparently in the prime of life and strong as horses, are suddenly carried off by cardiac infarction. The family, colleagues and the public are shocked by the catastrophe.

How can we explain what is nowadays the most frequent cause of heart failure, killing off healthy men of forty-five to fifty-five and women of sixty to seventy? The coronary vessels encircle the heart in the region of the waist between auricles and ventricles. From these arteries the heart is supplied and nourished with blood. Arteriosclerosis has a preference for afflicting just this much disputed area of blood vessels, when cholesterol (a fatlike substance) narrows their size. Small channels very easily form in the inner walls and eventually, like a cork, stop up one of the heart's blood vessels. With tragic suddenness an area of blood vessels essential to life is deprived of nourishment and with it the heart too—and the patient soon dies.

American research workers have found out in animal experiments that the so-called reticulo-endothelial system (certain cell areas in the spleen, the marrow of the bones, lymph glands and elsewhere) can, so to speak, filter out an excess of cholesterol in the blood. But one must beware of drawing wrong conclusions from this. It is known that female sex hormones strengthen the reticulo-endothelial system's work of lowering the level of cholesterol in the blood of the male organism. But injections of female sex hormones yield in exchange female sex characteristics in the male body. How can the one be achieved and the other avoided? The prompt and persistent action of the fast in lowering the cholesterol content is irrefutably proved. And what could be more suitable for making the good effect of the fast permanent, than a subsequent drastic curtailment of fatty food? One must, of course, remain consistent in taking at the most an ounce and a half of fat per day. This low-fat diet and the yearly health fast are the best preventives against the spectre of cardiac infarction.

From the rich store of their extensive experience with fasting patients suffering from heart and circulatory disorders, Grote and Zabel stress, as do Buchinger, sen., and Scheele, that the treatment celebrates a special triumph here. The attacks of angina pectoris cease. The sufferer can again walk longish distances without undue trouble and even climb stairs slowly. Pulse and heart action improve and the blood vessels dilate. The *intermittent* limp (contraction of the calf of one leg resulting from damage to the blood vessels) is reduced or even stopped. It was repeatedly observed that by a rigorous fasting treatment gangrene of the toes can be improved and occasionally cured.

Many people often talk conspicuously about their advanced age. There are those who regard growing old as a somenow unpleasant problem, and on the other hand those for whom it is a matter of pride. People do not admit the truth that they are growing old, and that they begin to be subject to this process as soon as they stop growing. Only two possibilities of dealing with it are at our disposal : to go forward with dignity (if we have really grown old) in the changed circumstances, for which we are compensated by greater maturity and experience of life. Or we can oppose the process of ageing which we consider to be advancing too quickly. But how? By means of the annual cleansing fast, avoiding tobacco and alcohol, eating fresh food with little salt and well chewed (Bircher-Benner), breathing deeply while out walking, sound sleep (early to bed!), and systematically breaking off the habit of worry. The latter is, of course, very difficult. The true philosopher is the first to succeed and also the genuinely religious person and the sanguine whose natural happy disposition meets this demand half way in any case.

If we are speaking of growing old, we immediately think of *arteriosclerosis* (hardening of the arteries). That isn't quite appropriate. For just as there are (less often, of course) octogenarians with quite elastic, almost youthful blood vessels, so there are also younger people who already show clear signs of arteriosclerotic processes.

Does the cause of ageing lie with the impregnation even of the tiniest branches of the blood vessels with calcium and fat-like substances, which make the vessels rigid, narrow, brittle and inelastic? Or with the drying-up of the production of the sex hormone? Or with the enzymes having become increasingly incapable of functioning? (Enzymes are substances acting biochemically as catalysts, which have a most decisive function to perform in the metabolic process of our body.)

Today we know that all the symptoms of old age we have spoken of are to be referred to disorders, impurities and faulty tensions in the sphere of the vital vegetative nervous system. In this system, which directs all automatically (therefore involuntarily) functioning events in our body, we must therefore see the controlling predisposition for our growing old. The increasing saturation of the whole bodily tissue with poisons of metabolism is, of course, to be held jointly responsible along with damage to the vegetative nervous system from nicotine in smokers.

The *arteriosclerotic impregnation of blood vessels* can, it is true, be loosened only in part by the remedial fast. But the wholesome changing of the tone of the vegetative nervous system and the freeing of the whole organism from the metabolic poisons bring about first-rate and lasting results. On the basis of our experience we can think of the remedial fasting treatment as an ideal means of rejuvenation. In the use of the vitamin body "Rutin" extracted from buckwheat we apparently have at our disposal yet a further possibility of improving the fragile state of the arteriosclerotic blood vessels.

The impregnation of the calcium-like platelets in the blood vessels is not a failure of the body, but the body's effort to help itself. For primarily the organism does not appear to want the arteries to become lax; it tries to strengthen the vessels by impregnating them with calcium. The brittleness of the vessels conceals within itself the danger of apoplexy. The escape of blood from small fissures in the vessels occurs practically always in the area of the brain. The reason for the special threat to this area probably lies in the fact that the greater use of the brain in man also leads to a special sensitiveness and strengthening of the circulation of the blood to this site. For the reasons already described above it appears plainly self-evident that the fast recommends itself both for preventing apoplexy and after it has occurred.

Homoeopathy can give excellent support to fasting, e.g. with *Arnica montana*, while masseur and physiotherapist make efforts to recover the ground lost to paralysis. The results of a combined treatment of that kind are surprisingly good.

CHAPTER FIVE

HIGH BLOOD PRESSURE

WHEN we develop high blood pressure (of non-renal origin), we are at first slightly inclined to be annoyed about it (and that sends it higher still!). We assess it as an irrational occurrence and a functional failure of our body. In fact, high blood pressure is an ingenious compensating and self-regulating mechanism. Different causes may be more or less clearly seen to act together in producing this disease. The blood pressure can rise for psychological reasons when we are "nervous" on account of constant anger controlled with difficulty or persistent anxiety. But whole sections of blood vessels can also be put into spasm and contracted by arteriosclerotic impregnation. Metabolic poisons retained and deposited in the body also sometimes cause a spasm of the vascular system; for that part of the vegetative nervous system which determines the narrowness or width of the blood vessels is slightly irritated by the impurities.

However, the segments of tissues lying beyond the contraction must still be supplied and nourished with blood, as otherwise they would of course perish. How does the wisdom of the "inner physician" now arrange it so as to overcome the increased resistance to the current due to the narrowing of the artery? The organism helps itself by a compensatory raising of the blood pressure, even if this ingenious regulation is only an emergency measure and is achieved at the cost of an added strain on the heart. Have we no reason at all, then, to be thankful to this silently and wisely operating power of self-regulation and to support it by a sensible approach in our mode of living? We see, therefore, that the reasons which lead to the rise in blood pressure are given with the actual disease, but the rise in blood pressure is not this disease itself. High blood pressure is rather to be considered as a favourable sign of the proper working of heart and circulation. Therefore, in general, tablets for lowering the blood pressure, injections and iodine waters are not suitable as the sole treatment. They even lead at times to the rupture of blood vessels (e.g. strokes). If by means of chemical action we release the calcium-like impregnations from the walls of the arteries and seek to make them elastic again, the lowering of blood pressure which this aims at is dearly bought. We know that the arteriosclerotic impregnations represent a protective measure taken for the strengthening of blood vessels which have become brittle. If we seek to clear them chemically without regeneration and strengthening of the vascular walls, the result is bound to be an increased fragility, and so a greater danger of apoplectic stroke. Often our mistake is, of course, to try fast-acting and convenient remedies. But their effect is all too often attended with danger and moreover is only temporary.

But what else is to be recommended to a patient with high blood pressure as to a heart patient? We have already learned from experience that the misuse of tobacco is highly injurious. Nicotine is harmful to the sensitive vegetative nervous system and causes severe spasms in the fine capillaries which are one of the important causes of high blood pressure. With a preference for attacking the heart, nicotine is responsible not only for disturbances of rhythm and function but also for constrictions of the system of coronary arteries. The consequence to the impaired heart circulation is angina pectoris, which consists in very painful attacks of cardiac anxiety. Nicotine can also lead to gangrene of the toes, even of entire extremities, and the "intermittent limp" which has already been mentioned.

Fasting and total abstinence from tobacco—that is the key to healing! If we attend to a special manner of living and eating (salt-free, with plenty of fruit and uncooked food), to instruction in breathing, physical exercises, and a sensible reduction of weight, we have been fortunate in looking after our regained health. The annual repetition of the fasting treatment may be looked forward to!

It may seem a paradox to many that the fasting treatment also improves *low blood pressure*. But after an initial further slight lowering of the blood pressure (due to the effect of fasting) it is almost always in the post-treatment period higher than it was to start with. That agrees with the well-known normalising action of the fast: too high and too low blood pressure are equalised in the same way.

It does not surprise us at all that not only a tendency to apoplectic strokes and thrombosis but also recurring phlebitis and *chronic inflammatory conditions* react well to fasting. The same, however, is true of *chronic middle-ear inflammations* without a recognisable tendency to heal and of plethora.

The so-called *"executive's disease,"* which is appearing today to an increasing extent, has its origin in nervous exhaustion from too heavy a load of work and worry. Doctors speak of the dangerous consequence of "stress." "Stress" is persistent cverburdening, unceasing strain, continual psychic pressure; our ability to bear and adjust ourselves to it finally succumbs in the shape of this illness. The vegetative nervous system is thrown off balance. To stay fresh and keep awake, coffee is regularly drunk as a "pepper-up." People smoke—so they think—to be able to calm their nerves. In short, one lives in a constant state of tension, worrying all the time and getting excited, without relaxing for good, ample periods of recreation. Finally, the afflicted person also develops chronic insomnia.

The first warning signs of the appearance of such a complaint are headache, a no longer manageable inner discontent and restlessness, weak concentration, and dislike of everything and everybody, accompanied by mild agitation and loss of one's sense of humour. Work which previously had the power to satisfy, indeed gave pleasure, now becomes a too painful burden. These are the first symptoms of which one should become mindful. If a break is not taken to recover, the second stage appears—anxious sensations of cardiac pain, felt especially at night, many kinds of disturbances of circulation, nervous outbreaks of sweating, attacks of giddiness, and so on. The third stage, which is quite alarming and finally compels the patient to ease off and seek medical treatment, is marked by fitful heart failure, high blood pressure, circulatory crises, angina pectoris, "nervous breakdown," or an apoplectic stroke. So now the continuous disregard of man's biological needs has taken its revenge. In the breakdown outraged nature *extorts* its right to rest and relaxation, which had long been denied to it. Unfortunately, however, the breakdown often enough has such serious consequences that a *complete* recovery is no longer possible.

CHAPTER SIX

SKIN COMPLAINTS

As a schoolboy I once read with astonishment in a newspaper
that a man with gas poisoning, whose lungs had already been
destroyed to a considerable extent, had still gone on living for
a long time. For the skin had taken over a large part of the
work of the lungs and therefore of the kidneys. A short time
after it said in the report of an accident that an unfortunate
person had had about a third of the surface of his skin
scalded. In general a person cannot survive the functional
loss of one-third of the skin.

These two reports gave me a great deal of thought at the
time. Evidently the skin is more than merely a covering which
surrounds the body. It is an organ which has certain tasks to
perform and the welfare of which depends on the state of
health of the whole body. Conversely the health of the whole
body and individual organs also depends on the condition of
the skin! In a skin complaint we shall immediately look for
primary causes in constitution or allergy, or for signs of
metabolic or infectious diseases. Dermatologists like to refer to
the "wonder" organ. For the skin is a sensitive end-organ of
the vegetative nervous system, as in the course of development
the nerve substance has come from the skin. It has a special
power of expression which frequently allows the doctor to
judge the inner condition of the body. The skin patient also
suffers psychologically as a "marked man."

The main group of skin complaints is eczema, psoriasis,
nettle-rash, oversensitiveness of the skin, a tendency to ulcers
and boils, and erysipelas. The usual skin specialist's skill is
mostly exhausted in the diagnosis and mitigation of the complaints. The results of treatment by applying ointments, tinc-
tures and irradiations are—for example, in psoriasis—
admittedly quite unsatisfactory. This seems to us, however,
not at all surprising, if we bear in mind that by such
measures the symptoms are influenced only externally. On the

other hand remedial fasting gets to the root of the trouble. No matter whether the cause is to be sought in constitution, in a condition of hypersensitiveness, in a disorder of metabolism or in an infectious disease, fasting supplies the key which almost invariably fits.

A doctor who has been able to gain experience for any length of time in a fasting establishment is sure to be opposed to the therapy of eczema and psoriasis. As a rule these skin complaints respond to the health fast, to the clearing attack upon the system. The fasting treatment is all the more successful the less the skin diseases have been rubbed and burnt into the skin and the entire organism with too many dermatological and radiological procedures, e.g. X-rays. They react best if they haven't been treated too much. Of course, it is necessary that within the next year or so two or three repetitions of the longer, strict treatment should be made. Even if complete success is not always achieved in the first treatment, the moist inflammatory places dry up, the itching (which at first is intensified) stops, the patches of psoriasis peel off; all affected places are reduced to their original limits, indeed most of them disappear altogether.

It is possible, however, that just here or there a small patch of eczema or psoriasis persists. That should on no account discourage and disappoint us. For the body always likes to leave itself open, according to its constitution and particular state of metabolism, a small safety-valve. Of such possible "safety-valves" there are, of course, several others, e.g. sweaty feet, a cold in the head. An ailing skin site which persists compels the patient not to relax his conscientious observance of a sensible mode of living and eating. Then one day this remnant, too, will have disappeared as the reward of such care.

With what remedies can we during the fasting treatment back up the healing of skin diseases? We find that the fasting person reacts especially favourably to homoeopathic medicines. In this especially sensitised state his constitution is got to grips with by high potencies, e.g. sulphur, formic acid, etc. Stimulating treatments with injections of the patient's own blood and urine can also be carried out to advantage. Shave grass (*Equisetum arvense*) is a soothing local application of service in the healing of eczema.

How many people suffer from "*skin impurities,*" greasy skin and pimples! While fasting an attempt can be made to banish these impurities by means of a wheat-bran bath. Take half a pound of wheat bran, seven ounces of oak bark, $3\frac{1}{2}$ ounces of mallow (*Malva silvestris*), $3\frac{1}{2}$ ounces of marsh mallow, $3\frac{1}{2}$ ounces of camomile flowers (*Flores Chamomillae*). First let the oak bark and the wheat bran boil, then add the other plants, let it draw for ten minutes, and pour the infusion, after straining, into the bath water not exceeding 100° F. or 38° C. A good scrubbing during the bath heightens the effect. After each bath a rubbing or gentle massage with a good mild vegetable skin-lubricant is to be recommended. Always scrub and rub towards the heart. If the greasiness of the skin is not completely removed by bathing and scrubbing, use gentle pressure in rubbing these places well in small circles with a pumice-stone, and follow this by lubricating as described above.

What must I now observe after the remedial fast so as to prevent a return of the skin complaint? The diet should, if at all possible, avoid spices and kitchen salt as well as pork and sausage. A gentle sprinkling with sea water or "Titro-Special" salt can take the place of kitchen salt. Let the food be uncooked, with plenty of fruit, and include plenty of roughage and a little albumen, and be predominantly alkaline, e.g. tomatoes, fruit, potatoes, carrots, grape-juice, milk. Regulate the bowels! Control the urge to eat more than necessary for satisfying hunger.

The remaining suggestions are well known: care of the skin (e.g. scrubbing with a dry brush), well-timed light and air baths, complete abstinence from alcohol and tobacco, and further treatment with suitable homoeopathic remedies.

CHAPTER SEVEN

DIGESTIVE AND OTHER DISORDERS

OF all *diseases of the digestive organs* constipation is the most widespread. A doctor often finds that those who suffer from it attach no special importance at all to this symptom. They consider a daily dose of laxatives perfectly normal. Others again consider it quite in order if they have a spontaneous bowel movement only once every second or even third day. As Bircher-Benner rightly says, we ought in the normal way to have a spontaneous bowel movement three times a day! Why? Let us think of meals : three times a day we "import," therefore, to put it crudely, we ought three times a day to "export" ! A multitude of diseases and nuisances have their origin in the bowels, in particular, headache, rheumatism, heart and kidney complaints, skin troubles, and often even the dreaded disease of cancer. The Arabs call the area of the stomach and intestines the "father of affliction"; the great research worker Metchnikoff exclaimed to his pupils : "Death sits in the bowels !" "For the many ills of the world, for dire emergencies, for marital discord, for gloom, accidents, suicides, business failures and political set-backs there is often nothing else to blame than *bad digestion*," stated the clinician Franz Penzoldt, who died in 1927. Chemically conserved, seasoned and lifeless food, with colouring matter, badly chewed and mixed with too little saliva into the bargain, "is the hot-bed on which the fruits of the doctor's consulting hours ripen" (O. Buchinger sen.). The vital healthy bacterial flora in the bowels degenerates. Abnormal fermentation and decomposition inflate the bowels, often cause colicky pains in the area of the liver, stomach or spleen, oppress the breathing, hamper the heart and displace it upwards. Very soon there begin rheumatism, headache, and a generally poor state of health. Now the pharmaceutical industry's many kinds of tablets are taken. These, however, throw the bacterial environment of the bowels right off the rails. Often there is no rest until the patient is on the verge of despair and ready for hospital. The bowels have become a much over-stretched, stopped-up bag of wind and faeces. The blood and tissue are continually poisoned by the bowels. The harm to the intestinal bacteria also in the end causes many kinds of disorders of the cutaneous nerves to set in (Vitamin-B deficiency)—a symptom frequent at a time when food is heavily processed and deprived of its natural values. Even the fasting person who does not suffer from constipation is most surprised to find how many old hardened deposits in pockets of the colon still come away from the bowels more than half way through the treatment.

What are we to do then? To begin with, an examination of the state of the bacterial flora of the bowels is necessary. After that—fasting! Careful colonic lavage, specially blended teas, homoeopathic medicines, and breathing and relaxation exercises for loosening the area of stomach and intestines. A day or two before breaking the fast we begin to line the bowels afresh, so to speak, with a healthy bacterial flora by taking capsules which are soluble in the colon and which are filled with the helpful bacterial occupants. They now create a "friendly atmosphere" again, colonise themselves, and help us to digest the wholesome food. To stay well we must take care of our intestines with food which is close to nature. (For dietary rules, etc., see page 61.) The sulfonamides and antibiotics (e.g. penicillin) act very injuriously on the condition of the bowels. But caution is also advisable against white (refined) sugar and sugar commodities. It can already be proved that a 3 per cent sugar solution checks and harms the vital bacterial environment of our bowels.

We live in an age which has rediscovered the connection between mind and body in disease. In particular, the stomach and bowels are very often the stage on which excitement, anger and all sorts of everyday tensions work themselves out, e.g. in the form of ulcers or constipation. So therefore the bowels also oblige us to strive for inner equilibrium. Natural laxatives, in case they are still needed, are: linseed (chew well!) and figs cut up and soaked (perhaps even swollen with soaking in vegetable oil). Often ripe (therefore not green) olives do good owing to their natural oil. But they must be vigorously washed beforehand. Hazel-nuts, Waerland whole-meal bread (from wheat, barley, rye and oats) and soaked prunes are spoken of very highly as a natural means of regulating the bowels, taking it for granted, of course, that they are well chewed.

In *ulcers of the stomach and bowels* a regular fasting treatment is generally not indicated; for them rather a recuperative, reassuring atmosphere, special natural diet (raw potato juices) and specialised medical treatment. The same applies mostly to gastritis. In spite of the often good results of the fasting treatment of diseases of the small intestine and colon, it is always only after accurate medical examination and advice that a decision can be made. If that isn't observed, the patient will not be spared surprises and disappointments.

In *bronchial asthma* remedial fasting acts to alleviate, loosen, and almost always to heal. Even allergic asthma, which is generally hard to influence, is often improved by the fast, which reduces the irritation. During the treatment, however, psychological guidance is of great importance, for almost all bronchial asthmatic conditions have a disturbing, indeed aggravating, psychic component. Successfully to come to terms with it means bringing the patient real relief. Homoeopathic remedies support the treatment; still more effective, however, is individual and correctly applied instruction in breathing. And so fasting, reasonable exercise in the fresh air, cheerfulness, and deep breathing are rungs on the ladder to recovery for the asthma sufferer.

By *allergy* are understood *symptoms of oversensitiveness*, of a partly innate, partly acquired kind. Not only bronchial asthma but also hay fever, nettle rash and many forms of weals belong to the allergic diseases. In these symptoms, too, remedial fasting in conjunction with homoeopathic treatment intervenes in a remarkably favourable way. The hypersensitivity of the organism to certain substances is alleviated. The symptoms of diseases are made more bearable.

In commenting on *diseases of the kidneys and urinary pas-*

sages we can keep essentially to the proposition of Otto Buchinger sen.: "The fasting person's urine heals its own passages." The body tries hard to shed gravel and also stones during the treatment. We find the same, too, with concretions in the gall-bladder. By means of a morphia syringe, however, the fasting director must sometimes intervene to ease the passing of the stone. Not only acute nephritis but also its chronic forms are wholesomely influenced by the long fast. In contracted kidney the fast acts to prolong life. Of course, only an experienced doctor can judge the result; for it is not a favourable sign if the raised blood pressure of the patient with contracted kidney will not drop under the influence of the long fast. But even here the fast improves the entire state of health. The accumulations of water in the tissues are diminished. In all cases of kidney diseases, however, a special diet is to be prescribed after the fast and employed for some time at least. Doses of certain homoeopathic medicines almost always have a very favourable action (*Plumbum metallicum, Arsenicum album*). On the whole it can be said that the remedial fast requires an exact diagnosis for diseases of the kidneys and urinary passages. According to the result, a medical specialist in fasting can begin and carry out an intended treatment.

The same is also true of the fasting treatment for *women's complaints*. The origin of conspicuous symptoms, e.g. haemorrhages, pains, swellings, menstrual irregularities, etc., must first be clarified.

The fasting treatment, however, develops the best effects imaginable, especially in *complaints of the change of life* and disturbances of menstruation. On account of the deficient production of ovarian hormones associated with obesity, many female patients visit a fasting sanatorium every year with success. Nevertheless the "wonder treatment" achieves much more still: the tendency to vomiting in pregnancy is alleviated, indeed often removed, as is the tendency to miscarriages. Experience teaches that benign tumours of the womb, as, for example, myoma, show in prolonged fasting a tendency to grow smaller. After fasting in menopausal complaints a diet as rich as possible in fresh food and low in salt and spices is to be recommended. At least it should be low in meat and include more acidophilous yoghurt or sour milk (at most about a pint spread over the day). Stimulants and luxuries like coffee, strong tea with no milk, nicotine and alcohol should be avoided. Once a week, as well, a not too hot bath (perhaps with pine-needles added) and a massage of the whole body with a brush are very pleasant and health-giving.

In the same way the regenerative treatment by fasting has a favourable action not only on the many chronic conditions of poisoning which derive from the misuse of medicaments, but also on the *consequences of chronic misuse of alcohol and tobacco*. The bitter "Facts about Alcohol" (Hoppe) are widely known, those about the insidious effects of tobacco, on the contrary, are still for the most part less well known. However, anyone who has already lost all strength of will through addiction to tobacco, alcohol or morphine can hardly expect substantial improvement or cure from the remedial fasting treatment.

In discussing the so-called nervous complaints we must now make special mention of *migraine and chronic headaches*, which in most cases react splendidly to simultaneous homoeo-pathic treatment and fasting. At the start of treatment one has this impression, until the disease reacts by flaring up once more. After that, however, the attacks occur almost without exception less often and are milder, frequently to be com-pletely cured after one or two repetitions of the treatment. Of course, a change in the mode of living and eating is a neces-sary condition. Anybody who, on returning home, makes the same mistake as before will also sooner or later again have relapses after the fast. The most effective homoeopathic remedies for the treatment of migraine are gelsemium, iris versicolor, digitalis or spigelia.

Similarly patients who suffer from *neuralgia, neuritis, nervous disturbances* of many kinds, as well as those who suffer from chronic insomnia often fast with success. Of course the latter have to reckon with an initial but temporary reactive

worsening of their insomnia; here, too, the support of homoeopathic remedies sometimes works wonders.

One hardly expects *neurasthenics* to be good fasting
patients. Nevertheless they generally fast better than one
thinks. If they, too, do not always fully lose their worrying
mental symptoms, these complaints are almost always moder-
ated. However, in many a neurasthenic, as above all in practically every true form of hysteria, the inhibited mental
structure appears to be a special kind of auxiliary stabilisation
created by the organism's inner state of emergency. This
dangerous equilibrium should not be disturbed by fasting. It
is quite indispensable that the doctor should also have a good
knowledge of human nature. Otherwise he will experience
great difficulties with serious forms of neurasthenia and true
hysteria.

As regards the *latent predisposition to cancer* the remedial
fasting treatment is the method of choice. Even after a timely
cure of cancer by an operation, one should, if there are no
contra-indications present, remove by fasting the still exist-
ing susceptibility to cancer. Above all, however, this is now
the last chance to avoid all indulgence in tobacco, for in the
tobacco tar (as was shown long ago) are contained cancer-
producing benzpyrene as well as anthracene, phenanthrene
and creosote. For the prevention of cancer we avoid as far
as practicable all food suspected to have coal-tar colouring
matter. Little can be added to that by the fasting specialist.

It needs no further detailed discussion to state the favourable effect of remedial fasting on the many separate and
combined forms of *glandular disturbances*; for fasting stimulates the conductor of the great orchestra of the glands and
glandular organs. Glands which are overactive are toned
down and again others which act sluggishly are stimulated
anew. In short, following the powerful law of compensation
in fasting, the organism strives to reharmonise the hormone
economy.

It may also be mentioned here that in general, patients
suffering from a *goitre* pressing forward behind the breast

bone, with difficulty in breathing, can come through the impending operation with an abundant fast.

Patients with *exophthalmic goitre*, however, form an exception. They are not permitted to fast.

Quite often one hears and reads of the necessity of so-called *spring treatments*. In late autumn and winter fewer opportunities are available to most people for plenty of exercise and deep breathing in the fresh air. People often sit in badly ventilated and overheated rooms. In short, light, air, exercise and deep breathing are absent. Metabolism suffers and is deficient in the so important excretory processes. But not only in all these points is there something wrong : as supplies of fresh fruit, salads and uncooked food are short there is now a lack of vitamins, minerals, and materials for growth. The result is a typical state of exhaustion such as we have already described in detail, fatigue, disinclination, little capacity for work, fits of depression, headaches, etc.

Here, too, it means remedial fasting! And then building up with fresh food rich in vitamins!

PART TWO

HOW THE FAST IS CARRIED OUT

CHAPTER EIGHT

HOW IS THE FASTING TREATMENT CARRIED OUT?

You have unpacked your suitcase in your room, washed off the dust and refreshed yourself from the exertions of the journey. A meal of fruit has been prepared for you. It, too, is a refreshment but also the first prescribed measure to begin the treatment.

At the start of treatment it is also appropriate that you find on the table in your room a small publication which contains the rules of the house. A pamphlet can, for example, be devoted to convincing you that these rules have been drawn up in your own interest and from ample experience of fighting for the goal of human recovery. The full text can be formulated something like this:

The patient undertakes on his arrival at the establishment the obligation to observe the rules of the house.

The success of the treatment depends on it!

The practitioner has the right and also—in the interest of the patient's recovery—the duty to dismiss on pain of immediately breaking off the treatment those who disturb or violate the routine, which has been tested for many years.

The cuisine and mode of life of the sanatorium should not be compared with what is customary elsewhere. All details of the life here belong to a well thought-out and specially arranged programme of work for the recovery and building up of sick people. To measure it by the standards of life in an hotel or private house testifies to a lack of understanding of what is achieved here.

The exception to the rule is also a remedial factor in a tried method. Anyone who does not see that clearly from the start and who lacks confidence in the treatment is out of place here! Remedial fasting is an heroic treatment. We ask you to bear the inevitable in a good spirit and with humour. Everything that happens is necessary for the treatment.

The many "dreadful orders, prohibitions and warnings" do not spring from the old-maidish hypochondria of a quack, but from the conviction of a specialist in fasting who has had a long experience of both successes and failures and the conditions upon which they depend.

1. Conversations about illness, hard times, financial and other worrying matters as well as about meals, break the atmosphere of healing and fasting. That is why they are to be left out among the circle of patients.

2. The sanatorium is by tradition no enemy of the radio, but only of the noise which the radio makes. Therefore, if the radio appears at all desirable during the remedial fasting treatment, have it on so softly that it can be heard only in the patient's own room.

3. Ignorance creates offenders. Don't forget : read literature about fasting !

4. A fasting establishment is not a sanatorium *de luxe*. All too worldly lavishness does not belong to the style of the time, still less, however, to the style of a fasting establishment.

5. In a fasting clinic the ban on smoking for patients and visitors alike is compulsory. Throughout at least the entire period of treatment neither coffee nor alcohol in any form whatever are to be taken. For both coffee and alcohol overload the liver—apart from other health disadvantages. And it is just the liver which has to perform the main work of detoxication and purifying. In short, anyone who drinks coffee or alcohol while the treatment lasts sabotages the success of his own cure !

6. Punctuality is politeness—unpunctuality is impoliteness !

7. Visits to the cinema and theatre, although not forbidden, interfere with the full efficiency of the treatment—as too much conversation and diversion in general go against the spirit of the treatment.

8. Between noon and 3 p.m. the midday rest is the rule in a fasting establishment. The fasting patients lie at this time in liver packs.

9. The length of treatment is determined by the practitioner after consultation with the patient in the light of the findings of the examination.

10. The immediate care and supervision during the treatment are arranged by the person in charge of the ward, who keeps in constant touch with the practitioner.

11. The lectures on health education topics are a part of the treatment like the fasting itself. Non-attendance reduces the value of the treatment and for this the practitioner cannot be held responsible.

12. The first three days of fasting (particularly in the first treatment) and the first three building-up days are often critical days. On these days do not go on any at all long excursions or car rides, etc. However, a walk may be taken, as desired, during the treatment for at least half an hour in the morning or afternoon.

13. Baths : Twice a week by special request a hot bath (not over 100° F. or 38° C.) is got ready by arrangement with the nurse. Swimming is not allowed while fasting. Splashing in water up to the knees only with approval.

Perhaps, as you take in the spirit and letter of the house rules you will also wonder why fruit is the first thing offered to you here. The *fruit day* not only flushes out quantities of fluid retained in the body; it also sees to it that the remains of the last meal left in the bowel of a person who afterwards fasts consists of fruit and not of more putrefactive food residues.

After the meal of fruit the nurse will come to you and ask you to be weighed. The *weight card* which is handed to you through the office, preserves as its first record your weight on beginning the treatment : your starting price, so to speak.

After the weighing the nurse goes with you to your practitioner. To him it is evident that your consultant whom you trust—recommended fasting treatment to you and that you agreed of your own free will. It is just as clear to him, however, that now, when things begin to get serious, the changed situation and the new surroundings could give rise in you to many doubts and fears. Probably on your first visit to the dining hall—during your meal of fruit—scraps of talk reached you from the next table. "Regulars" (who sometimes like to set up as experts and old hands in front of newcomers) were perhaps bandying about words and ideas which sounded strange if not uncanny in your ears: "Glauber's," "Roeder's," "crisis days," "liver pack," "recoil symptoms," and more of the same kind.

The practitioner, therefore, reckons throughout with the fact that, if you are visiting him for the first time, you could be afraid of your own pluck. You can be sure that everything that confuses and alarms you is to him relied upon down to the last detail. Just as there can be no depth psychologist who has not during his training been himself the object of a "didactic analysis," there is also no specialist in fasting who is not thoroughly familiar with all the techniques and symptoms of remedial fasting from his own experience of body, mind and soul. In addition, there is the wide experience which he can gather with his many patients and their similarities and differences. You may, therefore, be certain of his full understanding from the first moment of the treatment and throughout all possible difficulties that may subsequently arise.

To begin with, of course, he will examine you carefully. He carefully notes down a complete record of your medical history from childhood to this present hour of your meeting. In the physical examination he notes above all the condition and efficiency of your heart, investigates the size and sensitivity to pressure of your liver as well as the tactile findings of the organs in the abdominal cavity. An examination of the extremities, of your joints and the nerve reflexes closes the account with which your adviser provides himself of the state of your organism.

If after that you have any worries, fears or queries, you may lay them before him with the confidence of one who knows that he is in safe hands. In full reassurance and trust you then leave the consulting room.

On the following morning you are then charged with visiting the laboratory for the purpose of certain blood and urine tests. If necessary, an electrocardiogram is also taken of your heart activity. And so the first morning in the treatment establishment already provides "work" for you; however, this "work programme" is definitely over about midday with another visit to the practitioner. During the *first day of treatment*—the fruit day—you will make yourself more closely acquainted with the spirit of the place which is supposed to be the means of your recovery and which certainly will be too. The three meals of the fruit day consist—according to season—of apples, pears, oranges, figs, prunes, and the like. Of course, you are allowed to help yourself within self-imposed limits; yet in general not much more than two pounds of fruit is usually consumed during this day. Should thirst, contrary to expectations, appear, you quench it between meals exclusively with water.

As you no doubt belong to those who intend to complete their treatment "with rhyme and reason," you will have made yourself thoroughly acquainted in the course of the fruit day with the essential technical assumptions of the fasting treatment through observation or reading literature.

With all that you have even corrected wrong first impressions, or had them corrected—on the occasion of the midday visit to the practitioner. When you set foot in his consulting room for the second time, you found on your adviser's desk next to your medical history some notes about your special *plan of treatment*. This plan of treatment was entered on your weight card : it now says there, for example, that you are advised to fast for twenty-one days; also all other physical or medicinal prescriptions are noted on the weight card.

Twenty-one days! You need not be alarmed. Yesterday and today, you have made in the grounds of the sanatorium, the personal acquaintance of patients who are still enjoying the best of health on the twenty-first, twenty-eighth or even thirty-fifth days of fasting. They were lively and inspired, had no more pangs of hunger, and—as happens in many cases—expressed at the most a certain regret that the fasting days now soon had to be terminated. It will be just the same with you too. Besides, the well thought-out recommendation which imposes upon you a certain number of fasting days is not an inflexible command or compulsion. Should it turn out in the course of your treatment that a shortening or lengthening (the latter more often happens, as you can imagine!) of the period of fasting prescribed for you is advisable, then you can rely upon it that this adjustment in your condition is achieved in the proper manner under the trained eye of experience in fasting.

Arm yourself, then, with the "passport to fasting" of your weight card as with a talisman! Your practitioner's "visa" will be entered on it daily, so that you possess in black and white a document of particular value. The card is now your most important document. The course of every day is precisely marked down with directions for the nurse and for yourself too. We may remind ourselves with a smile that the cure is now "on the cards," so to speak. With the weight card lies a leaflet which gives the rules of the house again but this time in a more thoughtful form, so that you can again and again picture to yourself the therapeutic environment and its profound importance. At the same time it says what the patient should demand from his own inner being and should radiate on his fellow fasting patients for the promotion of the health and healing of all. The text can, for example, be worded as follows :

A fasting sanatorium has a therapeutic goal which is adjusted to the whole individual. If attention is paid only to the body and its functions and not to the mind and spirit, then an important element of recovery is left out. Therefore a calm, inwardly composed atmosphere is a requisite for the success of the treatment.

In patients' conversations the superficial, materialistic or sensational should not predominate. The negative, depressing and disturbing (which also includes all political matters and all comments on current affairs!) do not fit into the inner life of the house.

That is why we ask for understanding of the fact that there is no general radio reception here, that we do not encourage the need which many patients have to be busy and hard pressed as they are in their everyday lives, and that we emphatically ask patients to observe whatever creates and maintains the healing atmosphere. This is done only for the sake of the patients, who want to experience the effect of all that is wholesome on body, life, mind and spirit. We are neither an hotel with appropriate "guest service" nor a platform for the mutual confirmation of patients in those wrong impressions and faulty reactions of the inner life which here should just be overcome and cured. Worries, anxieties and needs of the individual and common destiny may be discussed with the practitioner or inwardly worked out in connection with the group consulting hour; they do not belong, however, in the remedial style of life and in patients' conversations. We will support

every patient who resists disharmonious influence by someone he is talking to. Inner composure, which no one should
allow to be disturbed, is a prerequisite for the success of
the treatment. Mutual support of the patients among themselves is again and again necessary in every respect. Anyone
who wants to be blest takes great pains to be a blessing
himself!

All things considered, the person who achieves his cure
here should break off relations with his everyday life (an
everyday life which has indeed made him ill!). Let him
make good use of the period of treatment, instead of pursu-
ing his fondness for criticism, sensationalism, dissipation,
pessimism, etc.

The fruit day is followed by the "*Glauber's day*." Johann
Rudolph Glauber, who discovered the salts named after him,
was an alchemist in the tradition of the great Paracelsus. The
fasting specialist, too, practises a certain kind of alchemy. It
is true that he does not turn lead into gold, but he is concerned with transforming the base material of his patient's
choked and burdened organism into golden health. At the
start of this effort comes the basic purification. That is why
he first just sweeps clean the inner surface of his patients'
organism with the help of the strongly purgative salts discovered by Glauber.

For this purpose you receive on the morning of the day
after the fruit day about an ounce and a half of Glauber's
salts in one and a quarter pints of warm water. It does not
taste particularly nice. That is why the maid puts a small glass
of fruit juice by the bottle of Glauber's salts. Each bitter sip
from the glass you can sweeten for yourself with a sip of
fruit juice.

After the repeated and powerful evacuation which the
Glauber's salts cause, you will assume that you should now
go through the ensuing days of fasting with nothing in the
bowels. That is, however, a mistake. The human gut is, you
see, not only made to absorb the nutritive value from our
foods and to propel the indigestible constituents with the

help of its worm-like contractions so as to eliminate them; it serves much more also—as does our skin—for excretion from the interior of the body, in which discharges take place through the intestinal wall into the intestinal canal. Furthermore, the organism retains for an unusually long time in the pocket of the colon faecal residues which are frequently a cause of inflammation of the mucous membrane.

Of that you yourself will immediately be convinced. The Glauber's salts have removed the residues which were present in the bowel. After this general cleaning out you get a cup of peppermint tea, so that the disturbance in the abdominal cavity is again quietened. No further food, however, is now given to you. The practitioner would not find it necessary to prescribe an enema every second day in the early morning for his patients if their bowels did not go on being filled by the "inner excretion." It may be surprising, however, for you to experience how up to the tenth, fifteenth or even the twentieth day of fasting the enema water still brings to light all kinds of intestinal contents.

After all, the fact is not quite so strange. Metabolism occurs, of course, even in the fasting organism. It may sound paradoxical but the fasting person "feeds on himself." He lives—although this is still to be accepted—on what is left to him; he metabolises the most impure and inferior material which is at his disposal (a process which O. Buchinger sen. named "refuse disposal" or "*burning of rubbish*"). Even as a convinced follower of vegetarianism one can say that a fasting patient's organism nourishes itself thoroughly on flesh, although it is the poorest which he can get hold off, namely, his own ailing or disease-ridden tissue. In this fast-conditioned form of "malnutrition" (which of course leads to an unequalled loosening) what cannot be decontaminated or eliminated by the air in the lungs or by skin or liver activity is discharged into the bowels.

You will, therefore, have to get used to an enema being introduced on every second day of your fast following the Glauber's salts. The fasting days pass off according to the following plan :

The enema referred to is followed by the drinking of a cup of peppermint or camomile tea. After that—if you have not been given an appointment in the consulting room— you can take it easy until 11 a.m. You can go for a walk or occupy yourself with your inner being in the quiet of your room. At eleven o'clock in the dining hall you get a glass of freshly pressed, clear fruit or vegetable juice or a cup of hot, clear fresh vegetable broth, in the evening, tea or sweetened grape-juice. The fresh juices or teas may perhaps not be to everyone's taste. But their aim is medicinal and they are to be measured by this scale alone. (If you get *too* thirsty during the day, you need not regret taking a quiet drink of fresh tap water, also certain mineral water, such as Pyrmont *Säuerling*. Indeed, if you want to be particularly successful in losing weight, then throughout some fasting days drink exclusively Pyrmont *Säuerling* or just pure, fresh, good spring water. That is a tested prescription for more vigorous weight reduction. Supplies of fluid must vary in kind and amount only within reasonable limits which are to be drawn individually in consultation.)

CHAPTER NINE

REST, EXERCISE AND HEALTH EDUCATION

FROM twelve o'clock to 2.30 p.m. *rest in bed* is prescribed for you. The Priessnitz hepatic binder which the nurse administers to you at this time powerfully stimulates the activity of your liver, for this detoxication centre in our metabolic laboratory has to work harder during the fast than in everyday life. You can already see from this fact, to which others like it can be added in plenty, that remedial fasting is not something passive while resting "far from the maddening crowd." The healing effects of the fast take place actively throughout. While your stomach, for example, works less, your liver works more and harder than in everyday life, when you change your organism over to fasting. That is why the liver is helped with the rest in bed as well as the *liver pack*, both measures aiming in the same direction. A human body at rest lays no claim— as does one actively moving about—to a more vigorous supply of blood to the muscles and brain; so the liver can, during the rest in bed, avail itself of an influx of blood not needed elsewhere. For this reason it is also recommended in daily life, through a short physical and mental rest after meals to afford the digestive organs an unrestricted and increased flow of blood. A fasting person's liver receives the desired influx of blood through the wet, warm pack, which is put on cold and then warmed by rubber hot-water bottles in accordance with a well-tried hydropathic method.

When the period of your rest in bed and liver pack is over, you must take care not to get up all at once but to do it restfully and gradually. The reason for that is clear from the one just discussed : the liver and, of course, the other adjacent organs in the abdominal cavity, when richly supplied with blood, are in possession of it at the expense of the brain circulation; if you now jump up from the horizontal position to the vertical, you are expecting too much of the speed with which the circulation has to adapt itself to a flow of blood newly brought back to normal. A feeling of giddiness, which in itself is irrelevant although inconvenient, a blackout, indeed in many cases a slight faint can be the consequence. For that reason take care here, too, in your own interest not to force your organism, for it is grateful for moderation, while it responds to compulsion with disturbance of its functions.

These and similar details (as well as matters of real importance) in the art of living will be explained to you in full in the lectures or group discussion periods, as we call them, which are held on four evenings a week and which I shall at once go into more closely. This work of enlightenment is an essential part of the fasting treatment.

You think about it best during your morning or afternoon walk, which is a part of the wholesome rhythm of the day's treatment. Just as during the midday rest it was the turn of

the liver for the strengthened supply of blood, which is
necessary for the correct functioning of all organs, so now it
is the turn of muscles and brain. When we go for a walk we
exercise practically all muscles in an ideal manner, not only
those of the legs and arms but also as a result of *deep breathing* those between the ribs and also the diaphragm, which
"massages" the organs of the abdominal cavity; we also use,
however, the important heart muscle and the millions of still
more important small muscles which cause the fine expanding
and contracting play of the capillary vessels of the blood
circulation. On the condition of the capillaries depends a
large part of the fate of our health; that is why—especially
in the biological aspect of medicine—a capillary diagnosis has
proved its value for the constitution. The walker, however,
also exercises his brain and—this time in a different sense
than that of a muscle—his heart. Not for nothing were great
philosophers of antiquity expressly "Peripatetics," that is to
say, they grew wise while walking about. In the morning or
afternoon walks which form part of your daily fasting programme you, too, should co-operate in the conscious percep-
tion of what the treatment is doing for you. Besides you can
again see that fasting has highly active principles. To begin
with, your will has been active in carrying out the treatment
according to instructions and in saying a spontaneous "No"
to food during the days or weeks which you will spend in
fasting. Again, during the period of fasting your "inner
physician" should be active—more active than in the normal
course of life. Finally, your consciousness should join actively
in everything that occurs with the renewing of body, life and
mind. This manifold activity can, however, take place only
while the inner being achieves silence and receptivity instead
of living continually in struggle and strife.

During the walk in the beautiful surroundings of the fasting sanatorium, chosen by you, you will perhaps pursue quite
by yourself thoughts like these :

"I am not fasting because I have for the moment lost my
appetite, but because I have resolved to do so of my own free
will. The alert will says no to meals during my period of

fasting, if the craving for them should be marked. Thus my human will is directed against one of the most commonplace of biological needs, against the desire to eat daily or several times a day."

If, as your practitioner hopes, a walk inspires you with these or related thoughts about what is a new kind of activity for you, then you have got the right attitude to anticipate something of the *religious mystery of fasting*. From remote antiquity down to the present day, healing and starvation have been more closely linked together than one commonly anticipates (although the leading brains of present-day medicine know and stress that already). Part of the phenomena of fasting can indeed be explained by the fact that lower realities are temporarily eliminated or held in check, so that higher realities can come to full realisation where otherwise too much of the lower disturbs and encroaches upon them. The highest reality, however, which can and will exercise beneficent sway in man is the Divine, from which all order proceeds—and ultimately all health. The time of fasting is a time of resting, because then man rises above the mundane into the sphere where the Divine gives renewal for body, mind and spirit. It also becomes clear to you, especially if you think of the very great part which fasting played in the early forms of the Indian, Persian, Hebrew, Christian and Mohammedan religion, that every fast is a remedial fast in the twofold sense of "divine service." On the one hand you serve as a person purifying himself in the fast, as one actually recovering divinity, while you restore the image of man which creation intended (for it intended the healthy person, not the sick, who is a distorted and darkened copy of the prototype). On the other hand the divinity serves you, too, as you fast, with all the powers of restoration which are now at work in you.

For the practitioner it is a particularly wonderful experience to see a good many of his patients becoming very quickly infected and inwardly fired by the *atmosphere* which a sanatorium filled with the proper spirit of healing should have. We have already witnessed many an inner transformation, many a fresh start of a human destiny and way of achievement which was already decided in the first few days of the treatment. Therefore, it is not unlikely that you, too, will find during your first or second walk, access to these innermost precincts of healing and salvation—in your own individual way, of course. And so you will come mentally and spiritually well prepared to the group consultation hours.

The lectures, the group consultation hours, as we call them, supplement the consultation hour in the course of which you daily confront your practitioner alone and consult with him about details of your special course of treatment. Every time there are enough personal matters to discuss. All that applies equally to everybody cannot be allowed to outweigh the personal and take up the time and energy of both parties. But that is not the only reason why on four evenings a week everything worth knowing and taking note of about the treatment is reported to the assembled patients by the practitioner. You must certainly all be instructed together about the fast itself, about details of the course of treatment, about the Röder procedure, homoeopathy, wholesome food, and so on. This happens systematically in the framework of the group consultation hours. However, the growth of a cure-promoting community atmosphere is more important still. Therefore the subject-matter of the lecture during the group consultation hours goes deep : it does not rest content merely with describing the treatment, explaining the measures and giving *training in the art of living*, but the more fundamental things of human life are generally discussed as well. You have the right to put written questions into a box which is placed at the entrance to the lecture room—and, as experience teaches, these questions relate only in part to the healthy, but more often they are questions about the way to find and realise the meaning of life.

In participating in these group consulting hours you will learn that the education for living which is to be attained thereby is of decisive benefit to you during and after the treatment. During the treatment, because this simply succeeds better and is of more real value if you yourself take part of your own free will and with genuine understanding. The person who only lets himself be forced through the period of fasting or taken in tow by the practitioner reduces the profit which he can and should have from this royal road of the healing art. Through the fact that you yourself are willing to cover the road you spontaneously induce the healing metabolism of fasting. You are then fasting as a whole person and not only as a passive object of solicitude.

When your first day of fasting and its conclusion, the lecture of the group consultation hour, are behind you, you have now already penetrated deeply into the nature, working and mystery of this treatment. You have also—partly in the form of direct instructions and partly through the content of the lecture—become familiar with technical details of the daily programme.

CHAPTER TEN

BODILY CARE DURING THE FASTING DAYS

THIS chapter is important to you and your state of health. You have already heard that the fasting person's bowel is switched to inner elimination. At the upper end of the alimentary canal, in the mouth cavity, the tongue offers a good example of such processes. When acting as an organ of elimination during fasting the tongue is thickly coated. Of course, an unpleasant mouth odour also appears; the fasting person's breath is bad. But what might appear to us abnormal in that is in reality the body's coping with its diseased substances. For what does a person live on while fasting? On himself! He is in a state of "autocannibalism," that is to say, he consumes human flesh—his own. The ailing tissues, the waste material and deposits of fat are first and foremost "digested." No wonder that with such "food" the organism is busy getting rid of the lower-grade material in any way it can.

4

Where refuse dumps smoulder and smoke as they burn to ashes, one cannot expect pleasant smells. That is why meticulous care of the mouth is necessary—just like the daily cleansing of the bowels by the enemas already described. Your practitioner also comes to your aid in dealing with the offensive smell. *The troublesome taste in the mouth and bad breath* make difficulties for every patient fasting—it has a downright unsocial effect on non-fasters. The detoxication and the cleansing inevitably involve that. It was Gustav Jaeger who said "Disease means stench!"

What can be done? It is right to distrust artificially compounded gargles, tablets and pastilles, and also the artificially produced chlorophyll preparations which are all the rage just now. Probably their activity does not stop at the physiological growth of bacteria in the mouth cavity but, where it is effective, also throws into confusion the normal proportions of bacteria by checking the general process of fermentation. What, then, will we recommend? Sips of natural lemon juice! Or a few peppermint lozenges each day—consisting of nothing but sugar and peppermint oil.

In every home for fasting patients a small herb garden should be available at the appropriate season. With lemon balm, chervil, thyme, parsley, chives or other herbs in small, finely-chewed quantities the mouth odour and taste can be corrected in a simple and inexpensive way. Thus we possess in chlorophyll, the green colouring matter of plants (which is moreover closely related to haemoglobin, the red colouring matter of the blood), an effective means of reducing the fasting person's mouth odour and bad breath.

You yourself have a means of increasing elimination and of "ventilating" the organism beneficially if you strive for

Cultivation of Vital Breathing.

It is well known to you that the individual life of man begins with the "first cry," a respiratory process, and ends with the "last breath." You know, too, that there is an innermost cell-breath and that besides the lungs, the skin also co-operates to a great extent in breathing. *Care of the skin in fasting*—washing, dry scrubbing, cautious sunbathing on prescription as well as *baths or physical exercises in the open air*,[1] and the like—increases the breathing of the skin and with it the combustion and elimination of what is diseased. Of special benefit, however, is the free breathing of the lungs, if you practise correctly. That goes without saying. The director of fasting will always make for himself a thorough selection of the best auxiliary methods which lie at hand. He wants neither to tempt you with breathing instruction to break records by performing like a bellows, nor to turn you into a yogi who breathes himself into mystical ecstasies. It is up to him to make the "divine breath," which in almost every ordinary person has become flat and cramped, a power contributing once more to their healing. With that you will notice that in any case while fasting you succeed in breathing more freely and easily. No wonder! For fasting removes one of the real obstacles to breathing, namely the inflation of the stomach and intestines. In an extraordinary number of people the diaphragm—that important elastic muscle which plays a main part in breathing—is forced up on the left side by a "football"—an air bubble at the top of the stomach. The stomach is inflated hard with wind (we find this particularly in unconscious "air-swallowers"). The colon, too, shows great gas bubbles which, as it is cramped, cannot escape. As a result the diaphragm is pressed upwards towards the heart—and the heart, which is therefore shut in, suffers pain. Many "heart complaints" (which can occasionally intensify into a symptomatic picture resembling angina pectoris!) are nothing but this pressure of gas, which can indeed "almost oppress the heart" of a person made ill by it. In

[1] Experience shows that Sauna and certain mineral baths can be combined with fasting under supervision for patients of sound heart and stable circulation. In certain female complaints *mud sitz-baths* can often with good results be combined with fasting (for disorders of the joints *mud packs*). P.T. in the morning, conscientiously carried out and well timed, has proved very effective, especially if it includes breathing exercises. While fasting one can seldom dispense with *massage of fibrous tissue* as little as with the thoughtful regulation of body movements in the form of walking. Technically blessed but poor, we human beings would certainly get along better if we walked more!

medical language this very common finding is called "gastro-cardiac syndrome" or Roemheld's syndrome after the physician who first described it. Roemheld had his patients literally breathe out these complaints by systematic breathing exercises for the diaphragm. On the other hand, as long as this syndrome is left untreated, especially by breathing therapy, it is a hindrance of the first order. As during the fast the "Roemheld cases" cease to be such, quite of their own accord, the fasting patients again breathe more and more freely.

Of course, it is by no means enough in all cases to remove mistakes of breathing. About the correct mode of breathing—which extends to close attention to the streaming in and out of the breath—the group consultation hour will have something important to say to you. It is also your practitioner's business in the personal consultation hour—drawing on breathing instructors and masseurs—to correct the particular mistakes of breathing of the individual case. That is important in numerous complaints. Asthmatics have altogether a wrong method of breathing. By spasmodic inhaling in the attack they fill their lungs too full, which in any case are filled with residual air, instead of emptying them first by a fear-dispelling deep exhaling. Every breathing exercise begins basically with deep breathing out. Whenever you hear of deep breathing, always bear in mind that deep breathing out is necessary. And if you ask whether one should cultivate chest or abdominal breathing, the answer can only be : full correct breathing penetrates into the deep region of the diaphragm (which stretches and protrudes the abdominal muscles a little by gentle compression of the organs in the abdominal cavity), and also fills the chest with its inrush. On breathing out the diaphragm is again lifted, the abdomen lowered, and afterwards the chest. Not only asthmatics, but all patients, in fact, are in need of such full breathing—which also prevents obesity. Heart patients in particular, however, need it. In angina pectoris freeing of the breath is incidental to the necessary auxiliary methods of successful treatment. The nervously excited heart can be calmed by breathing. The congested liver is freed from blockages by deep breathing. Cramps in the stomach and bowel area—also the very widespread painless spasmodic constipation—react most favourably to breathing therapy. The same is true of spasm-conditioned disturbances of circulation. Ide (Amrum) made use for a decade of systematic breathing therapy for the prevention of cancer. A host of disorders of the vegetative and central nervous system are favourably influenced by regulation of breathing. In particular, however, the restoration of free-flowing breath, which refreshes the organism in crampless fluctuating rhythm, stands the fasting metabolism in good stead. That is why general and, where necessary, special breathing instruction is one of our problems which is surely in great need of your co-operation.

While you therefore co-operate in the success of your treatment, your attention will also turn to the feature which strikes the layman most and which appears most desirable to the majority of fasting patients—weight reduction.

CHAPTER ELEVEN

LOSING WEIGHT

FASTING brings about a kind of "correct adjustment of the load," and so the curve of weight reduction can always be judged only individually. A person who puts on weight every year in the spring and summer of his life—body material mostly of the highest-grade waste—will get rid of far more than a less heavily loaded organism. *Abnormally thin people can also be allowed to fast*; they then take off only a little and at the end of their fasting régime attain a normal weight far in excess of what they started with. Research lacks precise scales for exactly assessing the degree of a person's total cleansing. We do not know, for example, exactly what is the state of juices and tissues in the probably long, latent preliminary stage from which cancer comes. We know only that cancer does not suddenly appear out of the blue—and we are

entitled, indeed it is our right and duty, to assume that the
inner situation of a precancerous organism is in particularly
urgent need of being purified and put right. Now the fasting
specialist again and again sees that in the one case a person
reduces "normally," i.e. as he usually does on the average; in
another case substantially less, and in a third, violently sudden
losses of weight can occur which appear to stand in no relation at all to the physical constitution and to the disease
picture of the patient concerned. Yet nature also speaks an
infallibly plain language.

In the third case, in which a person suddenly loses weight
at an alarming rate, it was obviously high time that he began
to fast, for his organism had a great deal of badness to get
rid of very quickly. Still it cannot be proved in such cases
that it is a question of precancerous symptoms, but it is getting
extraordinarily close to it. Quite definitely, however, the
position was serious, otherwise the curve of loss of weight
would have looked different.

If you think that over, you will understand *how absurd it
is to want to judge the results of the treatment only from the
scales.* One of the most annoying complaints to which the fasting specialist is exposed is a patient's envy—uttered in a
deeply offended tone—of the fellow patient who has lost more
weight. Every picture of disease is individual, no one position
at the start of treatment is like another—and from average
findings with regard to loss of weight you should never con-
clude that you, too, must naturally belong to the average.
In addition the loss of weight is, of course, more vigorous in
the first few days of fasting than later on. The fruit and
Glauber's salts days are already acting with a tremendously
dehydrating effect and in a manner which can be checked by
the scales. Among patients with abnormally swollen tissues
these days can cause a greater loss of weight than even the
succeeding days of fasting. Otherwise, however, the fasting
days are also apt to bring more vigorous loss of weight at first.
There is a most plausible reason for that. I will make it clear
to you by an analogy. In Canada and Alaska it happens that
outlying farms are cut off in the winter and fuel stocks run

low. At the same time, however, roads and railways are blocked by snowdrifts for long periods. The farmers now have to burn any unwanted furniture they can lay their hands on. First of all it is the turn of lumber which is accumulating dust : broken furniture, old magazines and books, all sorts of dust-traps, and in this way a "spring cleaning" takes places of necessity. If even then sufficient fuel for heating was not always obtained, the next step is to consider what can now be sacrificed for heating purposes. At last only in the most desperate cases will tables, chairs and beds also be put in the stove.

Something like this happens in the fasting organism. At first it is generous if no further food is given to it : it has, of course, more than enough to burn. The more inferior the material the less compunction there is about burning it in the fire of metabolism. Gradually, however, after deposits of fat, impurities and degenerated tissue have been consumed, the body substance can no longer be treated so generously. A kind of work with the chisel then commences. Everywhere that burdens and deposits are still partly to be done away with, without risk of greater losses, the delicate inner mechanism carries out work of amazing detail like a surgeon operating without a knife. In this phase dangerous and stubborn deposits are mostly attacked. Only if the hidden corners have been cleaned out, does the organism have to approach valuable remaining areas of flesh to maintain its metabolism while fasting. That, however, is the moment when the experienced practitioner terminates the actual fasting treatment and guides it over the breaking of the fast to the building-up.

You can see from all this that the reduction in weight is never exactly predictable, and that its comparison with another fasting patient's cannot be made. At a much earlier stage the individual loss-of-weight curve can permit a kind of "supplementary diagnosis," as it tells us about the diseased condition in which you began the treatment.

Therefore the scales every morning afford no measure of the success of the treatment. A fasting person who is in an optimistic mood will be pleased if he reduces relatively little, because he realises from this that he was burdened with relatively little dross—and he will also be pleased if he reduces a great deal, because that shows him how much he needed the treatment and how thoroughly it cleans him out and sets him up again.

Optimism, the belief in the best, the inner holding on to all that is wholesome is one of the powerful mainsprings of recovery. Optimism is the will to get well, expressed in a confidently positive psychological attitude. That has to do with something which cannot be weighed. In such important and decisive imponderables you should not let yourself be confused by the scales, still less when there are also other fluctuations in loss of weight which are quite simply conditioned by the treatment. For example, because you get no enema or liver pack on Sundays and holidays, on the following day the degree of loss of weight is apt to be less than usual.

If the check on your weight comes at the beginning of the fasting day, the visit to your practitioner follows immediately. There you also become acquainted with one of the auxiliary methods of the fasting treatment, called the "Roeder." The Elberfeld doctor, Heinrich Roeder, has worked out a method which by sucking and swabbing the tonsils and lower nasal passage has a wholesome effect on the mid-brain, the pituitary gland and the vegetative nervous system. O. Buchinger sen. was able to give this method a firmer basis and to build it up into an important auxiliary measure in fasting. He has stated the essentials of it in his book *Die Roedermethode* (Wilkens-Verlag, Hanover). Here let it only be revealed that the fasting patients come through crises more easily if they have had the Roeder treatment—and that the reason for it is to be seen without more ado. The tonsils have been considered by Roeder as an eliminating organ of the lymphatic system. Once let these filters be blocked—often by foul-smelling plugs, then one of the discharging outlets of the body is closed and it becomes a case of reintoxication. Hence the tremendously freeing action on the lymphatic circulation if the tonsils are repeatedly sucked by means of a small glass shade with a connected rubber tube and a suction ball. At the same time a

stronger flow of blood to these organs is achieved. In the lower
nasal passage are the end organs of the vegetative nervous
system which stand in reflex connection with organs of the
abdominal cavity, e.g. the gall bladder, stomach, duodenum,
womb, etc. A swabbing is like a good rousing knock which
calls these organs to order, so to speak. This applies especially to the tonsils, which function chiefly during childhood
and can then be sometimes abnormally enlarged, but in the
adult are preserved only as a small residual organ. It is an
important fact that developmentally the tonsils represent an
offshoot of the anterior lobe of the pituitary gland—the most
important part of one of our glands of internal secretion
which is closely linked with the mid-brain (as its "south pole").
A swabbing of the tonsils acts as a healing stimulus to the
higher centres. Therefore the Roeder action has an importance which we should not like to miss as an auxiliary method
to the remedial fasting treatment.

A further important auxiliary method, which has already
been gone into and should be gone into still further, is *the
patients' right mental attitude or their psychological healing
guidance by the practitioner*. Here let it just be said in this
connection that you must bring about such a right attitude for
your own benefit if crises and disturbances arise in the course
of the treatment. Complaints breaking out are mostly a good
sign. Your *reaction to fasting* is altogether desirable to the
practitioner and so it should be to you too. To him and the
experienced patient it is a familiar fact that often old complaints break out again in succession, like a film projected
backwards. In such critical phases the mood can be depressive.
That, however, can be avoided, indeed reversed, if the biological significance of such processes is really *understood*. In
about the last third of the treatment a mood of elation
prevails.

It shouldn't, however, put you in a bad humour to know
that during the fast you tend to *shiver* and *feel cold*. Visiting
the outdoor swimming pool is prohibited for this reason. For
the sudden considerable loss of heat in the cool bath can lead
to shock, disaster, or drowning. The heat necessary for the

combustion of your metabolic by-products is used up internally. This is yet another process full of significance. As the patient's organism becomes unusually sensitive he is more vulnerable to the effect of every stimulus than in everyday activity. It rests with you to keep from him stimulating impressions of a negative kind and to make the most of his vulnerability to wholesomeness, confidence, and to all that affirms the meaning of the treatment. Assistance—where necessary—is derived mostly from the healing treasure chest of Hahnemann's homoeopathy. Again and again we find that people whose capacity to react was practically defunct, e.g. as a result of misuse of medicaments or after X-rays or radiotherapy, recover while fasting the response of their organism to biological stimuli. So here there has been a particularly suitable field of operations for homoeopathy.

If in fasting the excretion of water becomes less than the requisite daily norm, that is seen to be favourably influenced by medicine from the golden rod (*Solidago Virgaurea*) and in actual heart weakness with *Cynosid compositum*. Do palpitations trouble you in fasting? The heart is working overtime the same as it was at the beginning of the treatment. But palpitations *are* troublesome! You are helped by *Crataegus oxyacantha* (from the hawthorn). For tense feelings of cardiac anxiety *Cactus grandiflorus* (perhaps even better the combined remedy of the homoeopathic "gold drops"). Excited sleeplessness with crowding thoughts as under the action of coffee, readily yields in fasting to *Coffea*. The disturbing but not very painful restlessness of the legs which prevents sleep disappears just as readily with a dose of *Zincum metallicum*. From these selected examples you can see how Hahnemann's homoeopathy is capable of correcting the fasting treatment as it is carried out.

CHAPTER TWELVE

HOW LONG SHOULD WE FAST?

THAT is now indeed the question. If there are no contra-indications for fasting, we can proceed by rule of thumb.

The more stubbornly chronic and the more anchored in the constitution the disease is, the longer the fast should last. Of course, the results of the examination and those of the laboratory must form the basis of our opinion. A fast should, if possible, last not less than fourteen days and we are hardly likely to go beyond a thirty-day fast. It is only seldom that the fast will be continued up to forty days. It rests with the fasting director's gift of observation, his experience and therapeutic ability to mark out here his field of action with the individual patient. His criterion is the patient's reaction and the result that can be attained. A written note is made of the duration of treatment. If necessary, changes are possible according to the way the treatment goes. The patient is aware that the plan can be modified.

Only the person of limited experience in fasting looks for objective signs in his own or someone else's organism, so as to be able, from the *signs of the so-called completed fasting state*, to finish at the right moment for breaking the fast. After forty, forty-eight and even fifty-two days of fasting the tongue can still be seen to be coated. Sometimes, too, the fur on the tongue disappears temporarily during the fast for reasons which are still not clearly understood—only to appear again. A fresh outer appearance, urine which has become clear or a return of signs of disease, etc., permit just as little a conclusion about the completed fasting state.

With the duration of fasting specified above, namely at least fourteen and if possible, twenty-one days, one can't go far wrong. The transition from fasting to hunger will be between about the fiftieth and sixtieth day of fasting. This transition consists in the fact that the disease and waste materials have actually been removed and now the fasting organism begins to melt down its own healthy tissues and organs. It will be practically impossible to settle the exact point of this transition from fasting to hunger. The longest fasting treatment which I have supervised from first to last was forty-two days. The case was a female patient who was seriously ill with high blood pressure and eye complaints. She throve on fasting and did not want to stop even on the forty-second day.

WHEN CAN THE FAST BE BROKEN?

This can be finally settled only by the fasting director's experience. Even under favourable conditions chance incidents can move us to break off the fast prematurely. For any particular reason (e.g. psychological or to do with the thyroid gland) the pulse rate can increase to more than 120 per minute. If it shows no sign of returning to normal we let the treatment be broken off with a simultaneous dose of aconite and tincture of Baldrian. Angina pectoris patients can still get an attack during the treatment (although usually they don't). The attack need cause no alarm and can be cleared by bathing under the arms with increasingly hot water; in that way the continuation of the treatment can be guaranteed. Then no more nitro-preparations are generally needed. In the fast there occasionally appear certain conditions which are caused by a fall in the level of blood sugar or calcium; they respond promptly and effectively to a small quantity of genuine turnip syrup dissolved in a mug of hot water.

We can now say that even a fool can fast, but only a wise man knows how to *break the fast properly and to build up properly after the fast* ! Whether the treatment will turn out a success or a failure is decided by conscientiousness in breaking the fast and by the method and diet of the building-up. Moderation in quantity and quality of the prescribed and supervised building-up diet is essential. The building-up period should be observed for at least seven and if possible fourteen days. In the building-up the fasting director can give his patient something like the diet plan and directions which follow in the final chapter.

CHAPTER FOURTEEN

DIET PLAN

Do you know that the most important building-up meals, the varieties of fresh food, lose in vitamin value ten minutes after preparation? For that reason be punctual for meals! Your punctual appearance adds your own health benefit to the gratitude of the hard-working kitchen staff. The quantity and kind of food and the compilation of the menus are the result of many years' experience and careful thought. The portions served are maximum quantities : they may be reduced according to how much the patient can eat, but on no account exceeded. The aim of the meal on a building-up day is not to become full! Many patients in the building-up stage eat at this time too richly for their own good, and still also occasionally (in town, in cafés, on excursions, etc.) the wrong kinds of food. That, of course, also includes coffee, cakes, pastries, whipped cream, etc. *All foods other than the ones given here are doubtful for patients who have completed a fast* and are therefore forbidden.

The return of the organism to healthy functioning must take place lovingly and in a sensible, progressive and moderate way. The rules of eating (eat slowly and in silence and chew each mouthful thoroughly) are never more important than just at this building-up time. The building-up days from breaking the fast onwards are, therefore, by no means a licence to return to the old mistaken ways of living, but they are at least for the coming weeks an after-treatment period calling for a sense of responsibility. Otherwise you jeopardise the success of your treatment.

It is emphatically a question of the building-up diet being *prescribed. No regard can be had to individual vagaries of appetite.* Justifiable objections to particular dishes or to the whole arrangement from the point of view of special health considerations are to be brought promptly to the practitioner's notice after the handing over of this diet plan.

From many years' experience the fresh apple has definitely proved the best way of introducing the breaking of the fast. Its organic trace materials are conveyed to the organism in the natural and undepleted form in which pectin and the core have a function promoting peristaltic movement. The apple is to be eaten unpeeled and the core as well. But it must be chewed most carefully! Should the chewing action of natural or false teeth not be enough, it can be grated at the table and taken in this form after being well mixed with saliva.

BREAKING THE FAST :

An apple. Another for the afternoon. Evening : plain potato soup.

1ST BUILDING-UP DAY (Have you read closely the above general introduction?) :

In bed: Prunes or figs (soaked in water).

Breakfast: "Four Winds" tea; muesli (cereals, cereal germ); three apples for the day (not to be eaten with meals, but as a snack *between* meals).

Midday: Fresh salad, raw prepared carrot, mashed potatoes.

Afternoon: Weak tea with milk, sugar or honey, crisp-bread and honey.

Evening: Fresh fruit (e.g. apple, banana or orange), one-third of an ounce of butter, Graham and crisp-bread, rose-hip tea.

Anyone who wants to keep his weight down does well to go easy on bread and butter. A person who suffers from insomnia or is slightly nervous does well to avoid black tea and instead order bramble-leaf tea, apple-peel tea or rose-hip tea. These home-made teas are digestible, indeed rather more health-promoting than black tea.

2ND BUILDING-UP DAY :

In bed: Prunes or figs (soaked).

Breakfast: Muesli, butter, Graham and crisp-bread, one cup of buttermilk, three apples and about twelve hazel-nuts for the day.

Midday: Salad, carrots in butter, unpolished rice, a small bowl of junket as a sweet.

Afternoon: Butter, crisp-bread, tea.

Evening: Mixed salad, Graham and crisp-bread, butter, cheese, rose-hip or lemon-balm tea.

3RD BUILDING-UP DAY :

In bed: Prunes or figs (soaked).

Breakfast: Butter, Waerland, Graham and crisp-bread, some jam, one cup of buttermilk, three apples and about twelve nuts for the day.

Midday: Large dish of uncooked food with some onions, two potatoes in their jackets, two-thirds of an ounce of butter, a pan of sour junket.

Afternoon: Crisp-bread, butter, honey, tea (weak).

Evening: Whole-grain porridge with fresh fruit (tastily prepared), junket with herbal seasoning, Graham and Waerland bread, two-thirds of an ounce of butter.

4TH BUILDING-UP DAY :

Early on the ward: Prunes or figs (soaked).

Breakfast: Muesli; Waerland or Graham bread, butter, honey, jam, one cup of buttermilk.

Midday: Raw carrots with fresh pickled-cabbage or green salad with fresh pickled-cabbage. Soup in the cup. potatoes and vegetables. Junket as dessert. Fruit and nuts for the afternoon.

Evening: Green salad or uncooked food, Italian salad with mayonnaise, Waerland and Graham bread with cheese and butter. Tea as desired.

5TH BUILDING-UP DAY :

First day on full board, modified according to season.

See weekly menus of the establishment.

Unpolished rice is recommended on purpose. With unpolished rice began our knowledge of vitamins, which has been decisive for modern nutrition research. The harmful practice of husking and bleaching the rice grain (the cereal grain too) to make it look as white as snow was the cause of millions of people, chiefly in Asia, succumbing to the most serious vitamin-deficiency diseases. Only the unpeeled and unbleached rice grain guarantees the full health value.

The breaking of the fast begins at midday with an apple, which is carefully chewed and mixed with saliva. If the apple has agreed with you, the real breaking of the fast is celebrated in the evening. A garland is placed round the plate of the person who is breaking his fast. By candlelight he receives his unseasoned, plain but tasty potato soup with small tender pieces of vegetable and herbs. Beside the plate he finds a document signed by the fasting director which solemnly confirms the number of days' fasting completed here.

The fast-breaker does well to retire to his room after this and rest in bed with a hot-water bottle. Here is the best opportunity to reflect on important thoughts and also—now at the latest—to make good resolutions about carefully observing the *rules of healthy nutrition*. These are: Don't eat too much; begin every meal with fruit, salad or uncooked food; eat slowly; chew your food and mix it well with saliva; don't drink during meals; eat in silence; enjoy every mouthful and stop as soon as the pangs of hunger are appeased. For it is not hunger which makes people fat, but the appetite which still persists after hunger is satisfied—the pleasure in food!

In the building-up days the patient's pleasure and interest in his return to work grow stronger and stronger. On about the seventh building-up day come the final examination and parting advice. With a renewed capacity for, and pleasure in, work the patient departs purified by the fast and with an individually planned régime for his future mode of living and eating in his pocket.